Rehabilitation Activities Profile

Rehabilitation Activities Profile

Manual and description

G.J. Lankhorst
F. Jelles
C.A.M. van Bennekom

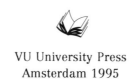

VU University Press
Amsterdam 1995

The Rehabilitation Activities Profile is developed at the Department of Rehabilitation Medicine of the University Hospital Vrije Universiteit with financial support of the Dutch Ministry of Welfare, Public Health, and Cultural Affairs.

VU University Press is an imprint of:
VU Boekhandel/Uitgeverij bv
De Boelelaan 1105
1081 HV Amsterdam
The Netherlands
Telephone (020) 644 43 55
Telefax (020) 646 27 19
ISBN 90-5383-398-6
NUGI 742

Design: Hans Jelles, Wormerveer

Foreword

In April 1991 the rehabilitation department of the University Hospital Vrije Universiteit in Amsterdam started a project which was entitled: *"Application of the International Classification of Impairments, Disabilities, and Handicaps* (ICIDH) *in rehabilitation medicine, a continuation study"*. The project was granted by the Ministry of Welfare, Public Health and Cultural Affairs and aimed at the development of an instrument to improve the quality and effectiveness of rehabilitation medicine. This novel instrument was called the Rehabilitation Activities Profile (RAP).

The RAP is guided by the concepts of disabilities and handicaps. Another important innovation is the integration of the subjective experience related to the disability or the handicap by the rehabilitee. This provides a central role for the rehabilitee in the RAP. In this edition the use and the individual parts of the RAP are described. An exact description of the used concepts is given, which should stimulate uniformity of language between the different rehabilitation workers. The RAP can be used also in different settings such as nursing home medicine.

We would like to thank all those who have contributed to the completion of the RAP for their support. We hope to have made a contribution to the quality development of rehabilitation medicine.

May 1995
G.J. Lankhorst
F. Jelles
C.A.M. van Bennekom

Contents

1 Introduction

In 1991 the rehabilitation department of the University Hospital
Vrije Universiteit in Amsterdam constructed the Rehabilitation
Activities Profile (RAP). The RAP facilitates the mapping of disabilities
and handicaps in the domains communication, mobility, personal
care, occupation and relationships.

History and background

In 1980 the '*World Health Organization*' published the '*Interna-*
tional Classification of Impairments, Disabilities, and Handicaps
(ICIDH)'. The ICIDH is a classification, which orders the consequences of disease. These consequences are specified on three levels
by the concepts impairments, disabilities and handicaps.

Impairment is defined as: "any loss of or abnormality of
psychological, physiological, or anatomical structure or function
(organ level)".

A disability is specified as: "any restriction or lack (resulting from
an impairment) of ability to perform an activity in the manner or
within the range considered normal for a human being (person
level)".

The concept of handicap is defined as: "a disadvantage for a
given individual, resulting from an impairment or a disability, that
limits or prevents the fulfilment of a role that is normal (depending
on age, sex, and social and cultural factors) for that individual (social
level)".

The ICIDH is no ready-made classification which can be
applied directly in each field, such as for instance rehabilitation. For
this purpose separate instruments have to be developed, based on
a selection from the ICIDH (*Wood, 1987*).

In the Jan van Breemen Institute in Amsterdam such an instrument was developed in 1988 and 1989. A list of 28 items were selected from the ICIDH, to register disabilities and perceived problems
related to these disabilities (*Jiwa-Boerrigter et al, 1990*). This
instrument is used mainly by physicians. Experiences with this
instrument provided the foundation for the Rehabilitation Activities
Profile (RAP).

In the construction of the RAP several disciplines have been
involved: rehabilitation physicians, physical and occupational therapists, speech therapists, social workers and psychologists of the
Jan van Breemen Institute, the Rehabilitation Center Amsterdam,
the St. Lucas Hospital and the rehabilitation departments of the

Academic Medical Center and the University Hospital Vrije Universiteit. All institutes are located in Amsterdam. In cooperation with these institutes the contents and descriptions of the items and sub-items have been defined and the RAP tried out in the clinical practice (*Bennekom et al, 1995a*).

Objective

The objective of the Rehabilitation Activities Profile is to document information on:
- the disabilities and/or handicaps in daily functioning of the person as result of disease, organ affection or accident;
- the perceived problem related to the disabilities and/or handicaps in daily functioning.

Rehabilitation medicine is aimed at enabling a person to function as independently and optimally as possible in his or her daily life. To make this goal concrete we selected those activities that represent this daily functioning as completely as possible.

In an interview with a rehabilitee, these activities are mapped by the interviewer, resulting in an individual profile of the disabilities/handicaps and related perceived problems.

Construction

The RAP consists of a list of activities and behaviors which cover five domains: communication, mobility, personal care, occupation and relationships. Each domain contains a number of items which are subdivided in sub-items. The RAP contains in total 21 items and 71 sub-items.

Scores are assigned to each item and sub-item, on four-point severity scales, concerning:
- the disability/handicap of the person on a certain item or sub-item;
- the perceived problem of the person with regard to the disability or handicap.

The RAP can be applied in multidisciplinary teams. For this application the items are assessed by the (rehabilitation) physician. This leads to the formation of the multidisciplinary team. Next, the other professionals make a detailed profile by assessing the sub-items of those items on which disabilities and/or problems were found. In principle a discipline is responsible for one or more items. In such a way each discipline has to fill in only a part of the list. This two-level structure reduces form-completion time on sub-item level and facilitates referral to medical and paramedical disciplines.

Reliability

Data concerning reliability of score assignment and completed score forms should be known before the applications outlined of the RAP are evaluated. The interviewer plays the most important role in score assignment and RAP applications. Therefore the reliability is defined by means of the inter-rater and intra-rater agreement (*Jelles et al, 1995*).

Several institutes and disciplines have been involved in the reliability study. The cooperation of the different institutes (rehabilitation centers and departments of university and general hospitals) have led to the involvement in the study of rehabilitees from different rehabilitation phases and from different diagnostic groups.

We distinguished eight diagnostic groups: rheumatoid arthritis; osteoarthrosis, post-traumatic disorders and other orthopedic disorders; amputation; low back pain, neck and shoulder pain (soft tissue disorders); cerebrovascular accident and other central neurologic disorders (excluding spinal cord lesions); peripheral neurologic disorders; spinal cord lesions; and remaining disorders. Inpatients as well as outpatients took part in the reliability study.

In the determination of the reliability of the items the physicians were involved, whereas the other team members were involved regarding the sub-items. The distribution of the 71 sub-items was made on the basis of the expertise of the discipline involved.

The study led to the conclusions that the inter-rater agreement as well as the intra-rater agreement concerning the score assignment on the items and the sub-items of the RAP is good to very good, provided that a good user instruction had taken place.

Validity

A validation study of the RAP as a disability index in stroke patients is performed (*Bennekom et al, 1995b*). The criterion, content, and construct validity of the four domains 'communication', 'mobility', 'personal care' and 'occupation' were evaluated.

Consecutive patients with a clinical diagnosis of stroke from four hospital departments of neurology were recruited for this prospective cohort study. In total 125 stroke patients who were still hospitalized on the 14th day after stroke were assessed with the RAP, the Barthel Index (BI) and the Frenchay Activities Index (FAI). Assessments were made at 2, 3, 4, 8, 12 and 26 weeks after stroke. The patients were visited at the hospital, at home, nursing home or rehabilitation center.

The domain 'mobility+personal care' correlated strongly with the BI score (r: 0.87-0.90) on all measurement points. The domain 'occupation' correlated with the FAI score before the stroke and 26 weeks after stroke (r: 0.72 and 0.73 respectively). The disability sum score of the combined domain 'mobility+personal care' allowed an accurate prediction of the living arrangement 26 weeks after stroke (Receiver Operating Characteristic area surface: 0.90). Mobility + personal care showed significant differences (p<0.05) in the eight-week disability sum score for the different living arrangements at that time: acute care hospital, chronic and intermediate care in a nursing home, rehabilitation center and living at home. Exceptions were rehabilitation center versus intermediate care in a nursing home (p=0.23) and acute care hospital versus chronic care in a nursing home (p=0.45). Hypotheses in mean score differences in the domains 'communication' and 'mobility+personal care' in subgroups could be confirmed (the subgroups were defined by: gender, having a partner, motor deficit of upper or lower extremity, urinary incontinence, higher cortical deficits, conjugate deviation of the eye, coma and hemianopsia, respectively).

It was concluded that the disability sum scores of the RAP can be used as discriminative, evaluative and predictive indexes.

Responsiveness

The responsiveness of the RAP and the Barthel Index (BI) was studied (*Bennekom & Jelles, 1995*). Responsiveness concerns the ability of an instrument to measure clinically meaningful change over time. Responsiveness was quantified using four techniques: effect sizes, p-values, t-statistics and Receiver Operating Characteristic curves (ROC). Having returned home six months after stroke was chosen as an external criterion.

The study population was the same as in the validation study (n=125). Three time periods were defined: 2 - 12 weeks (early response), 12 - 26 weeks (late response) and 2 - 26 weeks after stroke (overall response).

The effect sizes of the RAP were consistently higher in all three time intervals than those of the BI. Concerning the p-value techniques, the mean change score of the overall period of the RAP appeared to discriminate between patients returning home and not returning home, whereas the BI failed to discriminate (p-value .004 versus .496). Using t-statistics the RAP showed a higher efficiency in expressing change on the three time periods (Relative Efficiency: 1.42, 1.77 and 1.43, respectively). The ROC surface area of the RAP score was higher than the area of the BI score (0.74 and 0.59, respectively, for the early response period).

The conclusion was that all results indicated that the RAP is more responsive than the BI, when returning home six months after stroke is chosen as an external criterion.

Applications

The RAP may function as a communication instrument which structures the professionals' actions concerning people with disabilities and/or handicaps. The RAP can be used, for instance, for screening purposes, structuring communication between rehabilitation professionals and recording the severity of disabilities, handicaps and perceived problems for research or policy making purposes.

We studied two applications of the RAP.

I The construction of a predictive model using the RAP for returning home after stroke (*Bennekom & Jelles, 1995*).

Prognosis of stroke outcome is important to set realistic rehabilitation goals. A predictive model was constructed for the probability of being at home 26 weeks after stroke. The predictors found at two weeks after stroke for having returned home 26 weeks after stroke were also used in models predicting outcome at earlier stages (3, 4, 8 and 12 weeks).

The study population consisted of a subpopulation from the patient group of the validation study. Only patients with a supratentorial stroke were included. One-hundred-and-eleven patients were included in the study. The living arrangements of the patients were recorded 3, 4, 8, 12 and 26 weeks after stroke. Stepwise logistic regression was used to construct the predictive models.

The strongest predictors for being at home 26 weeks after stroke were (1) the sum score of the RAP domains 'communication', 'mobility' and 'personal care' at two weeks after stroke, and (2) age. Age was not a statistically significant predictor in the 3, 4, 8 or 12 week models after entering the RAP sum score. The predictive probabilities corresponded to the observed frequencies to a high degree for the 8, 12 and 26 week models, and to a lesser degree for the 3 and 4 week models.

It was concluded that functional status two weeks after stroke, as measured with the RAP domains 'communication', 'mobility' and 'personal care', enables accurate predictive modeling of being at home 8, 12 and 26 weeks after stroke.

II The process of structuring multidisciplinary team conferences with the Rehabilitation Activities Profile report system: RAP-TEAM (*Bennekom & Jelles, 1995*).

In this evaluation study two questions with regard to the Rehabilitation Activities Profile report system (RAP-TEAM) have been answered: (1) How does RAP-TEAM affect the satisfaction of professionals with team conferences? (2) What are the experiences of users with RAP-TEAM? RAP-TEAM has been introduced in three experimental teams in two rehabilitation centers. Seven teams in another rehabilitation center served as control teams. Questionnaires were used to answer both questions. Stepwise regression analysis was used to determine the influence on satisfaction of RAP-TEAM with as independent variables: gender, discipline, center, team, and social desirability.

A preliminary regression equation was drafted which expresses baseline satisfaction with team conferences. It was used for descriptive purposes only. Baseline satisfaction can be described with the equation: 3.73 + 0.64 physician + 0.03 social desirability + 0.40 control center - 0.69 team C7. Team C7 is a team in the control center. The constant value of 3.73 indicates that most professionals are neither satisfied nor dissatisfied with team conferences (score 3=rather bad, 4=neutral/no opinion). Being a physician increases satisfaction score by 0.64. Being a professional in the control center augments the satisfaction score by 0.40. Professionals in team C7 are less satisfied than professionals in other teams. Baseline satisfaction turned out to be somewhat influenced by social desirability.

The main regression equation to answer research question 1 uses the difference in satisfaction with team conferences as the variable of interest. Analysis revealed the regression equation: difference in satisfaction with team conferences = 0.15 - 0.90 team A1. Satisfaction had slightly increased in all experimental and control teams with the exception of experimental team A1. This means that RAP-TEAM had not influenced the satisfaction of most professionals with team conferences. Team A1 had become dissatisfied after introduction of RAP-TEAM. With regard to the second research question, it was striking that professionals report more benefits than disadvantages of RAP-TEAM.

The study report discusses several factors which would explain why in this study RAP-TEAM failed to influence satisfaction of professionals positively. The amount of time for introduction and adaptation seems to be a critical factor.

Literature
Bennekom CAM van, Jelles F. Rehabilitation Activities Profile, the ICIDH as a framework for a problem-oriented assessment method in rehabilitation medicine. Ph.D. thesis, Vrije Universiteit Amsterdam. Haarlem, 1995.

Bennekom CAM van, Jelles F, Lankhorst GJ. Rehabilitation Activities Profile, the ICIDH as a framework for a problem-oriented assessment method in rehabilitation medicine. Disability and Rehabilitation, 1995a, 17, 169-175.

Bennekom CAM van, Jelles F, Lankhorst GJ, Bouter LM. The Rehabilitation Activities Profile: a validation study of its use as disability index with stroke patients. Archives of Physical Medicine and Rehabilitation, 1995b, 76, 501-7.

Jelles F, Bennekom CAM van, Lankhorst GJ, Sibbel CJP, Bouter LM. Inter- and intra-rater agreement of the Rehabilitation Activities Profile. Journal of Clinical Epidemiology, 1995, 48, 407-416.

Jiwa-Boerrigter H, Engelen HGM van, Lankhorst GJ. Application of the ICIDH in rehabilitation medicine. International Disability Studies, 1990, 12, 17-19.

Wood, P.H.N. Maladies imaginaires: some common misconceptions about the ICIDH. International Disability Studies, 1987, 9, 125-128.

World Health Organization. International Classification of Impairments, Disabilities, and Handicaps: A manual of classification relating to the consequences of disease. Geneva: World Health Organization, 1980.

2 Interview

The RAP is interview-based. The key issue is whether the person actually performs an activity in daily living, not whether he or she is able to.

Information
In principle all information originates from an interview with the person concerned. The questions are asked directly to the person. Should the person be unable to answer adequately (for instance with an aphasic patient), a third person who knows the assessed person well can answer the questions. Information gathered through others (partner, family, nurses or therapist) can complete the profile. The goal is to obtain as complete a picture as possible of the disabilities and handicaps in daily functioning and the related perceived problems.

The RAP consists of activities which can be observed. It may be that observation by the interviewer or others leads to adjustment of the scores. In this way, possible observations in the consulting-room might be included in the score for a number of items or sub-items. Performance of activities or behaviors should *not* be provoked. In that case assessment will be of what a person is capable of doing and not what he or she actually does in daily life.

Period to be assessed
The questions are related to the week prior to the interview. After mutual consultation one can deviate from this.

Place to be assessed
The assessment of the items and sub-items will be based upon the activities in the daily living situation, in most cases the person's own home. However, in the clinical situation the assessment will be based on the person's activities within the (rehabilitation) clinic.

Interview structure
For each item or sub-item the interviewer first off all poses questions to get an impression of the degree of disability or handicap. For example: *"How do you manage to get dressed?"*, or *"Does it take you a long time to get dressed?"*

Next the perceived problem of the person in relation to the same item or sub-item is assessed. In this example one could ask: *"Does it bother you that you get yourself dressed with much difficulty?"* This sequence of questioning, first assessing the disability degree and then the perceived problem degree, has to be repeated for each item or sub-item.

From page 31 to 73 descriptions of the items and the sub-items are given for each domain, together with judgment criteria and example questions. The questions printed in italics should always be answered. One might proceed with the remaining questions. The interviewer is permitted to adjust the example questions to the person and the situation, and to ask supplementary questions. The example questions serve as an anchor point. Most questions mentioned in the manual are generally asked in the usual history taking.

Score forms

From page 75 the manual contains example score forms to note the scores. An empty line allows the scorer to make an additional remark on each score. In this manner an overall picture is obtained of the disabilities and perceived problems in daily living.

3 Guidelines for the score assignment

Disabilities are assessed in the domains 'communication', 'mobility',

'personal care' and 'occupation'. Handicaps are assessed in the

domain 'relationships'. The perceived problem will be assessed for

each disability and handicap. In certain situations an item or

sub-item might be not applicable or not judgeable.

Disabilities
How disabled a person is, due to a disease or disorder, can be
gathered from the daily life activities the person performs in his own
environment. In the RAP disabilities are discerned in the domains
communication, mobility, personal care and occupation.

The key issues of the interview are:
- does the person perform the activity?
- with how much difficulty is the activity performed?
- does the person receive help in performing the activity?

Disability severity grading
The disability severity grading comprises the aspects difficulty and
help.

The person performs the activity:
0 *without difficulty*
1 *with some difficulty*
2 *with much difficulty or with some help*
3 *not at all*

First, it has to be assessed whether the person performs the activity or
not. Performance means that the person fully performs the activity
him- or herself. Even supervision is treated as help from a person.
    If the person fully performs the activity on his or her own, the as-
sessment focuses on the amount of difficulty with which the activity
is performed (none, some or much difficulty). The concept difficulty
expresses how laborious an activity is for the person.
    If the person receives help from other people, the assessment
focuses on the portion the person actively contributes to the activity.
If this portion is substantial, severity grading 2 is assigned. If the
active contribution is entirely absent or minor, severity grading 3
is assigned.

Severity grading 2 incorporates the amount of difficulty as well as help from others. The reason for this is because difficulty and amount of help are often inversely proportional. For instance, the person might have much difficulty with performing a certain activity completely by him- or herself, but if some assistance (=help) is given, he or she performs it with some difficulty. In both instances severity grading 2 is assigned. One has to keep an eye on the active contribution of the person to the activity: does the person perform the greater part of the activity himself?

Assessment of the amount of difficulty
From page 31 to 67 the judgement criteria are described, to enable assessment of the amount of difficulty. The judgement criteria are the same for the item and its relating sub-items, with exception of the item *'professional activities'*. The criteria are worked out in the example questions. They form the anchor points for the interview and the score assignment. Most judgement criteria concern safety, speed, and the sequence of the constituting activities.

The assessor has to determine the amount of deviation from the 'healthy' population (the reference group). 'Healthy' population is defined as the group of people with the same age, gender, and socio-economic status (such as education, profession and living arrangement). The reference group will usually be formed by persons in the direct environment such as members of the family, friends/acquaintances and colleagues.

The assessment of the amount of difficulty in performance deals with the total impression of the interviewer on a certain item or sub-item. In general, the greater the deviation (in number or severity) of the reference group, the higher the severity grading.

Distinction between appliances and help
In the RAP 'help' is defined as help from other people. Supervision (for instance to ensure safety) comes under help. Although the use of appliances is not registered directly by the RAP, it could influence the severity grading. When the use of an appliance influences the performance, it will also influence the severity grading. The use of an appliance can be recorded on the score form on the empty line.

Practical instructions
The assessment of disabilities has to take place in neutral terms. First, the assessor asks whether the person performs the activity, for instance: *"Do you walk outdoors?"* or *"Do you cook?"*. Use of verbs like 'can' and 'able to' should be avoided. The RAP is aimed at assessing activities which are actually performed, not potential activi-

ties. Subsequently the assessor can ask: *"How do you experience walking?"*, *"How fast do you walk?"*, *"Do you have to rest?"*, *"Does someone accompany you?"*. Not until a total impression of the activity is obtained can the score be assigned.

Handicaps
The domain 'relationships' differs from the other domains because it stresses the social disadvantage. We have chosen to use the concept of handicap. The severity gradings of this domain differ accordingly. Instead of assessing the performance of the activities as such, changes in the activities are assessed.

Thus, what is assessed is the degree of change, due to the disease or disorder, which the person experiences in the continuation of his relationship with partner, child(ren) and friends/acquaintances. The content of the relationships before and after the manifestation of the disease is compared. Also in case of congenital or other longer existing disorders a change in health status will usually determine the patient's desires. In these cases changes in relations due to complications are assessed.

Handicap severity grading
The handicap severity grading expresses the degree of change.

Grading of handicap:
0   *no change*
1   *small change*
2   *large change*
3   *very large change*

The assessor has to determine whether the consequences of the disease brought about a change in the continuation of the relationship, as compared with before the disease or disorder. Only the impact of the disease on the relationship is assessed, not the content of the relation itself.

Assessment of the degree of change
The diversity of the sub-items has led to different judgement criteria for the different sub-items for the degree of change assessment (page 68 to 73). The criteria are worked out in the example questions to give anchor points for the interview and score assignment. Among other things, these concern frequencies of contact, disagreements and different task assignments. The interviewer has to assess to what extent these aspects differ from the situation before the disease or disorder. The reference group of the domain *'relationships'*

is the individual situation of the person concerned. The focus is on the relationships chosen by the individual and the contents given by the individual. We have chosen the person as his or her own reference because of the variety on behaviors within relations. This precludes referring to certain norms or habits.

Disagreements of earlier date concerning relationships are in principle not assessed. Latent discord may become manifest in a relationship as consequence of a disease. It is up to the interviewer to decide whether and to what extent such discord should be assessed.

The total impression is involved in score assignment. In general, the more the aspects change, in number and in magnitude, the higher the handicap score.

Practical instructions
The assessor has to pose questions in a neutral way. For instance: *"Has the relationship with your partner become different after your disease/accident?"* or: *"Have the consequences of your disease caused a change in the care for your children?"* Subsequently the assessor can ask in what respect the relation has changed. After obtaining a complete picture, the assessor can assign a score.

Perceived problems
The existence of disabilities or handicaps is mostly not sufficient for a rehabilitation indication. The perceived problem of a patient has to be taken into account.

The term 'perceived problem' is defined as the individual experience related to the disability/handicap in daily life. In other words, it is the amount of hindrance or bother the person experiences as a result of the disability/handicap. This will strongly be associated with the meaning of the activity for the person. The degree of perceived problem will be defined on the one hand by the degree the disability/handicap hampers the person in reaching certain goals in life or endangers these goals, and by the degree of adaptation on the other.

Perceived problem severity grading
For all domains the same score definitions are applied.

Grading of perceived problem:
0 *none*
1 *light*
2 *moderate*
3 *severe*

Assessment of the degree of perceived problem
There are no judgement criteria given in the RAP manual concerning the perceived problem scoring. The reason for this is that these aspects are strongly related to the individual. Guidance here is limited to a general directive:

0   No problem. The person indicates that the disability or handicap causes no problem in daily life. The life goals are not endangered.
1   Light problem. The person indicates that the disability or handicap causes slight problems in daily life, but these problems are surmountable and do not endanger the life goals seriously.
2   Moderate problem. The person indicates that the disability or handicap causes serious problems in daily life. The problems are difficult to surmount and seriously endanger the life goals.
3   Severe problem. The person indicates that the disability or handicap causes very serious problems in daily life. These problems are nearly insurmountable and attainment of life goals is hardly possible.

The severity assessment is performed by the individual patient. The interviewer assigns the scores on basis of the problem description by the patient. Thus the reference group concerning perceived problem is in all domains controlled by the norms or habits of the individual.

Practical instructions
After determining the disability/handicap score, the assessor has to find out, in neutral terms, about the degree of perceived problem. This can be done by presenting the four-point severity scale to a person and asking for a score indication. Also the assessor can ask questions like: *"Are you bothered by getting dressed with some difficulty?"*, or *"Are you hindered by getting dressed with some difficulty?"*.

Even more than with the assessment of disability or handicap, one should avoid questions that might influence the person's answer, like : *"You probably don't mind that you scarcely walk outside?"*, or: *"You must be bothered by needing help to cook meals?"*

It could happen that a disability assessment can be performed, but not a perceived problem assessment (for instance, in a severely aphasic person). In this case, one should assign the score 3 for the perceived problem.

Not applicable or not judgeable
In certain situations it may not be possible to assess the disability or handicap. Activities may not be applicable to a person or there may

be too little information available to make an assessment. Consequently, 'not applicable (NA)' and 'not judgeable (NJ)' can be assigned to the item or sub-item.

NA and NJ relate to the disability/handicap score as well as to the perceived problem. In the case of a disability or handicap which is not applicable or not judgeable, the perceived problem is not assessed.

Not applicable
When a person does not perform a certain activity, score 3 has to be assigned. However, if activity is not performed because the item or sub-item concerned does not apply to the person, the score NA is assigned.
This can happen in two situations:
1 The person forms part of the population for whom certain activities are not applicable.
   For instance:
   – the person moves from place to place by walking; thus the item *'using wheelchair'* is not applicable, or
   – the person has no partner; thus the assessment of the relation with partner is not applicable.
     This situation generally happens only with the items *'using wheelchair'*, *'professional activities'*, *'partner'* and *'child(ren)'*.

2 The person does not perform the activity, not because of the disease or disorder, but because someone else has made it his or her task.
   For instance:
   – the person does not clean the house, not because of his disorder, but because the partner always does the cleaning.
     This situation generally arises only with the items *'household activities'* and *'providing for meals'*.

In the second situation a professional judgement has to be made on the relation between the activity in question and the disease or disorder.
   When an activity is not performed, it might in some cases be difficult to determine whether either 'not applicable' or score 3 'does not perform activity' should be assigned. If there is a relation with the disorder, score 3 is assigned. If the relation is absent or unclear, one should ask whether the patient perceives a problem in not performing that certain activity. Should the patient perceive no problem, the

score 'not applicable' is assigned. If the patient does perceive a problem, the disability score 3 is assigned and then the degree of perceived problem should be assessed. Thus, in case of doubt, the person concerned decides whether the item or sub-item is applicable to him or her.

Not judgeable
Situations can arise in which there is insufficient information, verbally or by observation, to decide whether a person does or not perform a certain activity. In this case NJ (not judgeable) is assigned. For instance:
- in the early phase of rehabilitation not much is known about the relation with the partner or child(ren) to make a judgement on the score, or
- in cases of severe communication disabilities and no proxies or observations are available.

In theory, not judgeable can be assigned for each item or sub-item. In practice, it is seldom the case that nothing is known about the person's activities.

The assessor should strive to replace the score NJ as soon as possible with a score assignment of the disability or handicap.

4 A case

A fictitious case is presented to yield further insights into the score assignments. Only relevant facts are given in the case. Usually these facts are embedded in a more comprehensive history taking. The information is displayed in two profiles.

Personal details

Mary B., female, aged 44 years, was admitted to rehabilitation center K. on January 22, 1993. Medical diagnosis: large media infarct left hemisphere (December 26, 1992). Medical history: blank. Married, mother of three children (9, 11 and 13 years old), works part-time in a bookshop and lives in a single-family dwelling.

Admission (January 22, 1993)

Mary is dependent in activities of daily living. She manages to eat and drink reasonably well, although she needs help with cutting bread and meat. Transfers take place under supervision to ensure safety; the same applies to standing. Mary overestimates her capabilities in these and ignores problems. She only walks during the physical therapy sessions, with assistance of the physical therapist. She has not practiced stairclimbing yet. She would like to, because at home she has to climb the stairs to her bedroom and the bathroom. She manoeuvres with the wheelchair quite well inside; she has already learned this in the hospital. There are some serious communication problems. Mary understands everything, but has serious wordfinding impairments. This makes her feel desperate. She sleeps uneasily despite medication. She complains a lot about this. She washes herself almost independently, but needs assistance to wash her back and hair; she does not seem to be bothered by this. She gets dressed and undressed on her own, but takes up a lot of time doing so. "I have plenty of time", she says. Toiletting is supervised and she needs a hand now and then; this bothers her a bit. She is an enthusiastic participant of pastime activities, but is not able to do a lot. Her great wish is to leave the rehabilitation center on foot; she found the wheelchair transportation a nightmare. She worries a lot about keeping house when she returnes home. Her husband is very interested in the therapy and she gets lots of visits from her children and friends.

One month after discharge (April 25, 1993)

Mary has returned home. She manages quite well with the help of friends. She is still troubled by some slight wordfinding impairments. She manages to walk inside the house reasonably well; she rarely goes outside the house and certainly not on her own. Stairclimbing is difficult. Rising from a chair is troublesome; she has not regained her standing balance. At home she sleeps like a baby, without medication. Eating and drinking is going well with some assistance with cutting and buttering. Washing and getting dressed take more time than in former days, but she manages. Getting undressed is no problem at all. She manages toiletting with all sorts of tricks, she says. All these inconveniences does not concern her: "I simply have to accept it, there is no choice". Her biggest concern is the housekeeping and looking after the children. A girlfriend moved in to lighten these tasks a little for Mary. This person also sees to the daily meals, Mary can only give some directions in shopping and cooking. The girlfriend also keeps the house clean; Mary does some light housekeeping activities. She would very much want to do it herself. She comes up short with her children, she says: "few trips, they have to help me instead of the other way round". Emotionally she has still a good contact with them. She describes her relation with her husband as good; maybe their feelings have even deepened as a consequence of all the problems. She is not yet interested in taking up her hobbies. She gets a lot of visits from friends and neighbors: "Luckily they have not forgotten me". She often rides along with someone to visit friends. She has not been to the bookshop so far, as she does not feel up to it.

Rehabilitation Activities Profile

Items of all domains

Name : ...Mary B.. Date of birth : Nov. 11, 1949 Gender : m /(f)

Address : .... Diagnosis : CVA middle cerebral art. left

t-code/zip code : ....

City : .... Date : Jan. 22, 1993

Communication

		Disability	Problem	
• Expressing	:	2	3	....
• Comprehending	:	0	0	....

Mobility

		Disability	Problem	
• Maintaining posture	:	2	0	..overestimates!................................
• Changing posture	:	2	0	..overestimates!................................
• Walking	:	3	3	..only during therapy sessions............
• Using wheelchair	:	0	0	....
• Climbing stairs	:	3	3	....
• Using transport	:	3	0	....

Personal care

		Disability	Problem	
• Sleeping	:	1	3	..with medication..............................
• Eating and drinking	:	1	0	....
• Washing and grooming	:	2	0	....
• Dressing	:	1	0	....
• Undressing	:	1	0	....
• Maintaining continence	:	2	1	..supervision..................................

Occupation

		Disability	Problem	
• Providing for meals	:	3	3	....
• Household activities	:	3	3	....
• Professional activities	:	3	0	....
• Leisure activities	:	2	0	....

Relationships

		Handicap	Problem	
• Partner	:	N	J	..lots of visits................................
• Child(ren)	:	N	J	..lots of visits................................
• Friends/acquaintances	:	N	J	..lots of visits................................

Disability severity grading:	Handicap severity grading:	Perceived problem severity grading:
0 = Without difficulty	0 = No change	0 = None	
1 = With some difficulty	1 = Small change	1 = Light	
2 = With much difficulty or with some help	2 = Large change	2 = Moderate	NJ = Not Judgeable
3 = Not at all	3 = Very large change	3 = Severe	NA = Not Applicable

Rehabilitation Activities Profile

Items of all domains

Name : Mary B.
Address :
Post-code/zip code :
City :

Date of birth : Nov. 11, 1949 Gender : m /(f)
Diagnosis : CVA middle cerebral art. left

Date : April 25, 1993

Communication
(Disability / Problem)

- Expressing : [1] [0] ....
- Comprehending : [0] [0] ....

Mobility
(Disability / Problem)

- Maintaining posture : [1] [0] ....
- Changing posture : [1] [0] ....
- Walking : [2] [0] walking outdoors poor
- Using wheelchair : [N] [A] ....
- Climbing stairs : [1] [0] ....
- Using transport : [2] [0] ....

Personal care
(Disability / Problem)

- Sleeping : [0] [0] without medication
- Eating and drinking : [0] [0] ....
- Washing and grooming : [1] [0] ....
- Dressing : [1] [0] ....
- Undressing : [0] [0] ....
- Maintaining continence : [1] [0] ....

Occupation
(Disability / Problem)

- Providing for meals : [3] [3] by girlfriend
- Household activities : [2] [3] by girlfriend
- Professional activities : [3] [0] does not feel up to it
- Leisure activities : [3] [0] does not feel up to it

Relationships
(Handicap / Problem)

- Partner : [1] [0] positive
- Child(ren) : [2] [3] ....
- Friends/acquaintances : [1] [0] positive

Disability severity grading:
0 = Without difficulty
1 = With some difficulty
2 = With much difficulty or with some help
3 = Not at all

Handicap severity grading:
0 = No change
1 = Small change
2 = Large change
3 = Very large change

Perceived problem severity grading:
0 = None
1 = Light
2 = Moderate
3 = Severe
NJ = Not Judgeable
NA = Not Applicable

Description of the items and sub-items for each domain

The items and sub-items of the Rehabilitation Activities Profile are described for each domain. The domain is indicated on the top right of each page. Top left on each left-hand page the item at issue is indicated. Below this the item and its sub-items are described. The example questions are always printed on the right page.

Expressing

Item description
'*Expressing*' comprises the person's ability to generate and emit a message to another person (orally, in writing and/or using gestures and signs).

Sub-item description
- Nonverbal
  The conveyance of a message by means of sign-language, sounds (no words), mimicking, pointing, indicating yes/no, drawings or symbols.
- Talking
  The oral communication of a message: spoken language.
- Writing
  The written communication of a message: written language.

Criteria for judgement
  - Comprehensibility:
    form (audibility);
    content.
  - Suitability to the situation.
  - Level:
    limited to indicating yes/no;
    only concrete (everyday) topics;
    abstract topics.
  - Situational lack of freedom.
  - Time needed.
  - Perseverance in talking.
  - The degree to which the interviewer must assist the person, posing extra questions or guessing (this is considered as help of another person).

Questions
- Nonverbal

Does the person uses gestures, symbols or drawings?
  - Is the message understandable?
  - Does the message relate to the situation?
  - Does the message consist of only yes/no, everyday topics or also more abstract topics?
  - Does the person need a certain situation (surroundings or person) to emit the message?
  - Does the person need a lot of time to emit the message clearly?
  - Does the person get tired?
  - Is it necessary to assist the person, to guess or to stimulate?
- Talking

Does the person talk?
  - Is the message understandable?
  - Does the message relate to the situation?
  - Does the message consist of only yes/no, everyday topics or also more abstract topics?
  - Does the person need a certain situation (surroundings or person) to emit the message?
  - Does the person need a lot of time to emit the message clearly?
  - Does the person get tired?
  - Is it necessary to assist the person, to guess or to stimulate?
- Writing

Does the person write?
  - Is the message understandable?
  - Does the message relate to the situation?
  - Does the message consist of only yes/no, everyday topics or also more abstract topics?
  - Does the person need a certain situation (surroundings or person) to emit the message?
  - Does the person need a lot of timc to cmit the message clearly?
  - Does the person get tired?
  - Is it necessary to assist the person, to guess or to stimulate?

Comprehending

Item description
'*Comprehending*' comprises the comprehension of information by the person in contact with the surroundings or another person (images, sounds, nonverbal, spoken or written language).

Sub-item description
- Images
  The comprehension and recognition of images (objects, faces and situations).
  Excluding: sign-language, mimics, drawings and gestures.
- Sounds
  The comprehension and recognition of sounds.
  Excluding: spoken language.
- Nonverbal
  The comprehension of information expressed in sign-language, mimics, sounds (no words), pointing, indicating yes/no, drawings or symbols.
- Spoken language
  The comprehension of information given orally: spoken language.
- Written language
  The comprehension of information expressed in the written language: reading.

Criteria for judgement
- Form:
  word comprehension;
  sentence comprehension.
- Level:
  limited to yes/no or short simple words;
  only concrete (everyday) topics;
  abstract topics.
- Situational lack of freedom.
- Time needed.
- Perseverance in talking.

Questions
- Images

  Does the person comprehend/recognize images (objects, faces)?
  - What is the degree of recognition?
  - Does the person estimate distances well?
  - Does the person need a lot of time?
  - Does the person get tired after a short time?
- Sounds

  Does the person comprehend/recognize sounds?
  - What is the degree of recognition?
  - Does the person relate the correct meaning to certain sounds?
  - Does the person need a lot of time?
  - Does the person get tired after a short time?
- Nonverbal

  Does the person comprehend gestures, symbols or drawings?
  - Does the person need a lot of time?
  - Does the person need a certain situation (surroundings or person)?
  - Does the person get tired after a short time?
- Spoken language

  Does the person comprehend the oral message of another person?
  - Does the person comprehend only yes/no and short simple words, everyday topics or also more abstract topics?
  - Is there word comprehension as well as sentence comprehension?
  - Does the person need a lot of time?
  - Does the person need a certain situation (surroundings or person)?
  - Does the person get tired after a short time?
- Written language

  Does the person comprehend written messages?
  - Does the person comprehend only yes/no and short simple words, everyday topics or also more abstract topics?
  - Is there word comprehension as well as sentence comprehension?
  - Does the person need a lot of time?
  - Does the person need a certain situation (surroundings or person)?
  - Does the person get tired after a short time?

Maintaining posture

Item description
'Maintaining posture' comprises the active maintenance of the posture during activities by the person.

Sub-item description
- Lying
  The maintenance of the lying posture during the performance of activities.
- Sitting
  The maintenance of the sitting posture during the performance of activities and shifting one's position. Assessment is made of the chair, sofa, wheelchair or alternative transport in which the person mostly sits.
- Standing
  The maintenance of the standing posture during the performance of activities performance.

Criteria for judgement
- The safety during the performance of an activity in the lying, sitting and standing posture.
- The time span of the maintenance of a posture.
- The frequency in which a posture is maintained.

Questions

- Lying

Does the person actively maintain the lying posture during activities?
  - How safe is the performance of activities in the lying posture?
  - Does the person maintain the lying posture during a long time, if necessary for certain activities?
  - Does the person maintain the lying posture several times a day, if necessary for certain activities?

- Sitting

Does the person actively maintain the sitting posture during activities?
  - How safe is the performance of activities in the sitting posture?
  - Does the person maintain the sitting posture during a long time, if necessary for certain activities?
  - Does the person maintain the sitting posture several times a day, if necessary for certain activities?

- Standing

Does the person actively maintain the standing posture during activities?
  - How safe is the performance of activities in the standing posture?
  - Does the person maintain the standing posture during a long time, if necessary for certain activities?
  - Does the person maintain the standing posture several times a day, if necessary for certain activities?

Changing posture

Item description

'*Changing posture*' comprises the active change by the person concerned from one posture to another, for instance from the sitting position to the lying position. Also transfers are seen as a change in posture and are thus assessed under this item.

Sub-item description

- From lying to lying (lie/lie)
  Turning around in lying posture, like turning in bed from prone to supine and the other way round.
- From lying to sitting and from sitting to lying (lie/sit)
  Rising from the lying to the sitting position and lying down from the sitting position. This sub-item comprises different ways to change from lying to sitting and the other way round, for instance as well from supine to sitting with straight legs as from supine via lying on the side to sitting on the edge of the bed.
- From sitting to standing and from standing to sitting (sit/stand)
  Changing from sitting to standing and sitting down from the standing position.
- From sitting to sitting/transfers (sit/sit-transfers)
  Changing from one sitting position to another, as happens in moving or sliding from a wheelchair to a stair or from the (wheel)chair to bed. If the person first has to change to the standing position, take a few steps and then sit, this is not assessed under this sub-item. In this case the sub-item '*sit/stand*' is applicable.

Criteria for judgement

- The safety during the posture change.
- The time needed to change posture.
- The sequence of changing posture.

Questions
- From lying to lying (lie/lie)
  Does the person turn in the lying position?
  - Does the person turns safely?
  - Does the person need a long time to turn around?
  - Is the sequence of actions during the turning around correct?
- From lying to sitting and from sitting to lying (lie/sit)
  Does the person change from lying to sitting?
  - Does the person change from lying to sitting safely?
  - Does the person need a long time to change from lying to sitting?
  - Is the sequence of actions during the change from lying to sitting correct?

  Does the person change from sitting to lying?
  - Does the person change from sitting to lying safely?
  - Does the person need a long time to change from sitting to lying?
  - Is the sequence of actions during the change from sitting to lying correct?
- From sitting to standing and from standing to sitting (sit/stand)
  Does the person change to the standing position from sitting?
  - Does the person change to the standing position from sitting safely?
  - Does the person need a long time to change from sitting to standing?
  - Is the sequence of actions during the change from sitting to standing correct?

  Does the person change to the sitting position from standing?
  - Does the person change to the sitting position from standing safely?
  - Does the person need a long time to change from standing to sitting?
  - Is the sequence of actions during the change from standing to sitting correct?
- From sitting to sitting/transfers (sit/sit-transfers)
  Does the person change from one sitting position to the other?
  - Does the person change from one sitting position to the other safely?
  - Does the transfer take a long time?
  - How is the sequence of actions during the transfer?

Walking

Item description
'Walking' comprises the movement of the person by means of walking.
Excluding: the climbing of stairs. This is assessed under the item *'climbing stairs'*.

Sub-item description
- Indoors
  Walking indoors. This sub-item assesses how the person deals with factors like thresholds, doors, furniture, floor-covering and suchlike.
- Outdoors
  Walking outdoors. This sub-item assesses how the person deals with factors like pavements, obstacles like cars, weather conditions, noise, natural terrain and suchlike.

Criteria for judgement
- The safety during walking.
- The walking pace.
- The time span of walking.
- The frequency of walking.
- The distance covered.
- Taking short rests.
- The time of day during which the person walks.

Questions
- Indoors
  Does the person walk indoors?
  – Does the person walk indoors safely?
  – What is the walking pace like?
  – What is the time span of walking indoors?
  – How often does the person walk indoors?
  – Does the person get everywhere in the house?
  – Does the person take short rests?
  – Does the person walk indoors at every moment of the day when he or she wants to?
- Outdoors
  Does the person walk outdoors?
  – Does the person walk outdoors safely?
  – What is the pace like?
  – What is the time span of walking outdoors?
  – How often does the person walk outdoors?
  – Does the person take short rests?
  – Does the person walk outdoors at every moment of the day when he or she wants to, in spite of weather conditions?

Using wheelchair

Item description
'*Using wheelchair*' comprises the moving of the person, when this is performed with a handdriven or electrically driven wheelchair. *Excluding*: climbing stairs or slopes. This is assessed under the item '*climbing stairs*'.

Sub-item description
- Indoors
  The use of a wheelchair indoors. This sub-item assesses how the person deals with factors like thresholds, doors, furniture, floor-covering and suchlike.
- Outdoors
  The use of a wheelchair outdoors. This sub-item assesses how the person deals with factors like pavements, obstacles like cars, weather conditions, noise, natural terrain and suchlike.

Criteria for judgement
- The safety while using the wheelchair.
- The pace while using the wheelchair.
- The time span of using the wheelchair.
- The frequency of using the wheelchair.
- The distance covered.
- Taking short rests.
- The time of day at which the person uses the wheelchair.

Questions
- Indoors
  Does the person use the wheelchair indoors?
  - Does the person use the wheelchair indoors safely?
  - What is the pace of using the wheelchair like?
  - What is the time span of using the wheelchair indoors?
  - How often does the person use the wheelchair indoors?
  - Does the person get everywhere in the house?
  - Does the person take short rests?
  - Does the person use the wheelchair indoors a every moment of the day he or she wants to?
- Outdoors
  Does the person use the wheelchair outdoors?
  - Does the person use the wheelchair outdoors safely?
  - What is the pace of using the wheelchair like?
  - What is the time span of using the wheelchair outdoors?
  - How often does the person use the wheelchair outdoors?
  - Does the person take short rests?
  - Does the person use the wheelchair outdoors at every moment of the day when he or she wants to, in spite of weather conditions?

Climbing stairs

Item description
'Climbing stairs' comprises the bridging of all sorts of differences in heights, like stairs and slopes that a person has to deal with in daily living. The item is applicable to walking persons as well to those who use a wheelchair.

Sub-item description
- Indoors
  The bridging of a difference in height, like stairs to a higher or lower floor. The use of a (stair)elevator can also be assessed under this item.
- Outdoors
  The bridging of a difference in height outdoors, like stairs, a wheelchair ramp of a public building or the approach to a bridge.

Criteria for judgement
- The safety during bridging differences in height.
- The time span of bridging differences in height.
- The frequency of bridging differences in height.

Questions
- Indoors
Does the person bridge differences in height indoors?
  - Does the person bridge differences in height indoors safely?
  - How long does the bridging take?
  - How often are differences in height bridged?
- Outdoors
Does the person bridge differences in height outdoors?
  - Does the person bridge differences in height outdoors safely?
  - How long does the bridging take?
  - How often are differences in height bridged?

Using transport

Item description
Using transport comprises the movement outdoors of the person by means of transport (bicycle, car and suchlike).
Excluding: the use of a electrically driven wheelchair. This is assessed under the item *'wheelchair'*.

Sub-item description
- Bicycle/moped
  All factors related to moving oneself by means of a bicycle/tricycle and/or a moped. This concerns mounting and getting off the moped/bicycle and the actual riding.
- Car
  All factors related to moving oneself by means of a car. This concerns getting into and out of the car and the actual car driving. Also the use of other vehicles permitted on a motorway are to be assessed under this item.
- Public transport
  All factors related to moving by means of public transport. This concerns getting into and out of the vehicle and the actual travelling (like deciding on destination, places to change and suchlike). Public transport includes tram, bus, subway (metro systems), taxi, train, boat and suchlike.
- Alternative transport
  Moving oneself by means of transport not defined by the other sub-items. This concerns mainly low speed vehicles. Assessment is made of all factors related to driving by oneself by means of these vehicles. This concerns getting into and out of the vehicle and the actual driving.

Criteria for judgement
- The safety during driving and getting into and out of (or on and off).
- The frequency with which the means of transport is used.
- The distance covered.
- The time of day at which the person uses the means of transport.

Questions

- Bicycle/moped
  Does the patient ride a moped/bicycle?
    - In a safe way?
    - Does the person use the moped/bicycle as often as desired?
    - Does the person arrive at every place he or she wishes to?
    - Does the person use the moped/bicycle at every moment of the day he or she wishes to?
- Car
  Does the patient drive a car by him- or herself?
    - In a safe way?
    - Does the person drive the car as often as desired?
    - Does the person arrive at every place he or she wishes to?
    - Does the person use the car at every moment of the day he or she wishes to?
- Public transport
  Does the patient travel by public transport?
    - In a safe way?
    - Does the person travel by public transport as often as desired?
    - Does the person arrive at every place he or she wishes to?
    - Does the person travel by public transport at every moment of the day he or she wishes to?
- Alternative transport
  Does the patient drive an alternative means of transport?
    - In a safe way?
    - Does the person drive the vehicle as often as desired?
    - Does the person arrive at every place he or she wishes to?
    - Does the person drive the vehicle at every moment of the day he or she wishes to?

Sleeping

Item description
'*Sleeping*' comprises falling asleep and sleeping on.

Sub-item description
- Falling asleep
  The act of the person falling asleep.
- Sleeping on
  The person continuing to sleep.

Criteria for judgement
- Safety during sleeping.
- The time it takes to fall asleep.
- The time span of sleep.
- The frequency of sleeping.

Questions
- Falling asleep
Does the person fall asleep?
  - How long does this take?
- Sleeping on
Does the person continue to sleep?
  - What is the safety like during sleeping (for instance, with regard to falling out of the chair or bed)?
  - How long does the person sleep?
  - Does the person wake up often?
  - Does the person sleep several times a day?

Eating and drinking

Item description
'Eating and drinking' comprises both the preparation of food and drinks such as pouring out, serving and cutting, and the actual eating and drinking.
Excluding: cooking meals and making drinks. This is assessed in the domain *'occupation'* under the item *'providing for meals'*.

Sub-item description
- Preparing food
  The preparation of food and drinks just before eating or drinking, for instance: buttering and spreading of bread, serving, cutting, and pouring out.
- Conveying food to mouth
  The conveying of food or drinks to the mouth.
- Chewing/swallowing
  The chewing and the swallowing of food and drinks.

Criteria for judgement
- Safety of eating and drinking.
- Sequence of eating and drinking.
- Speed of eating and drinking.
- Efficiency of eating and drinking.

Questions
- Preparing food
  Does the person prepare food and drinks?
  - In a safe way (i.e., is there any dangerous use of cutlery, spilling hot fluids)?
  - In the right sequence?
  - How long does this take?
  - How efficiently (i.e., does the person spill drinks, cut too big portions)?
- Conveying food to mouth
  Does the person convey food and drinks to the mouth?
  - In a safe way (i.e., is there any dangerous use of cutlery, spilling hot fluids)?
  - How long does this take?
  - How efficiently (i.e., does the person spill food/drinks, eat only part of the food)?
- Chewing/swallowing
  Does the person chew and swallow food/drinks?
  - In a safe way (i.e., does the person put too big portions in the mouth, or does he or she chew insufficiently)?
  - How long does this take?
  - How efficiently (stuffs food/drinks in the mouth, drops food or spills drinks)?

Washing and grooming

Item description
'*Washing and grooming*' comprises the preparation of the washing and grooming (such as picking up and getting of soap, washing-glove and comb ready), as well as the actual washing, wiping off, grooming and putting away of washing or grooming materials. The applications of cosmetics is also included. No distinction is made between washing at a sink or a shower.

Sub-item description
- Face and hair
Assessment is made of the washing and grooming of the head. This also includes the preparation for that purpose and the subsequent putting away of the washing and grooming materials. This sub-item comprises the neck as well. The washing concerns hair, face, ears, neck, the cleaning of dentures and suchlike. Grooming concerns combing and hair-drying, shaving, applying after-shave, make-up and suchlike. The cleaning of contact lenses and glasses is also assessed under this sub-item. Factors like opening and closing taps, handling soap, washing-glove, shampoo, and so on are also assessed under this sub-item.
- Upper part of the body
Assessment is made of the washing and grooming of the upper part of the body. This also includes the preparation for this purpose and the subsequent putting away of the washing and grooming materials. This sub-item concerns the upper extremities and the upper part of the trunk. Grooming concerns cutting nails and applying nailpolish or varnish and rubbing in bodylotion. Factors like opening and closing taps, handling soap, washing-glove, shampoo, lotion bottle and so on are also assessed under this sub-item.
- Lower part of the body
Assessment is made of the washing and grooming of the lower part of the body. This also includes the preparation for this purpose and the subsequent putting away of the washing and grooming materials. This sub-item concerns the lower extremities and the lower part of the trunk. Grooming concerns cutting nails and applying nailpolish or varnish and rubbing in bodylotion. Also hygiene during menstruation, such as inserting tampons or applying sanitary towels, are assessed. Factors like opening and closing taps, handling soap, washing-glove, shampoo, lotion bottle and so on are also assessed under this sub-item.

Criteria for judgement
- The safety of the washing and grooming.
- The pace at which one washes and grooms.
- The result of the washing and grooming.

Questions
- Face and hair
  Does the person wash and groom his/her head?
  - Does the person wash and groom his/her head safely?
  - How long does the washing and grooming of the head take?
  - What is the result of the washing and grooming of the head?
- Upper part of the body
  Does the person wash and groom the upper part of the body?
  - Does the person wash and groom the upper part of the body safely?
  - How long does the washing and grooming of the upper part of the body take?
  - What is the result of the washing and grooming of the upper part of the body?
- Lower part of the body
  Does the person wash and groom the lower part of the body?
  - Does the person wash and groom the lower part of the body safely?
  - How long does the washing and grooming of the lower part of the body take?
  - What is the result of the washing and grooming of the lower part of the body?

Dressing

Item description
'Dressing' comprises the preparation of dressing (like taking and getting clothes ready) as well as the actual dressing.

Sub-item description
- Upper part of the body
  Assessment is made of the preparation of clothes for and actual dressing of the upper part of the body. This concerns the head, the upper extremities and the upper part of the trunk. This sub-item assesses the putting on of a blouse or a sweater, gloves, a hat and so on. The kind of clothes may influence the score. For instance, the person puts on summer-wear quite easily but needs help with a heavy winter-overcoat.
  Excluding: the closing of fastenings. This is assessed under the sub-item *'fastenings'*.
- Lower part of the body
  Assessment is made of the preparation of clothes for and actual dressing of the lower part of the body. This concerns the lower part of the trunk and the lower extremities. This sub-item assesses the putting on of pants, panty-hoses, shoes and so on. The kind of clothes may influence the score. For instance, the person puts on pants quite easily but needs help with a panty-hose.
  Excluding: the closing of fastenings. This is assessed under the sub-item *'fastenings'*.
- Fastenings
  Assessment is made of the closing of fastenings. This sub-item assesses zip-fasteners, bra-fastenings, boot-laces, buttons and suspenders.
- Body-worn aids
  Assessment is made of the preparation and applying of body-worn aids like splints, orthoses and protheses. Also the handling of glasses, contact lenses and dentures are assessed under this sub-item.
- Ornaments/adornments
  Assessment is made of the preparing and placing of ornaments or adornments like rings, chains and watches.

Criteria for judgement
- Safety during dressing.
- The sequence of actions during dressing.
- The speed of dressing.
- The result of dressing.
- Adjustment to the different seasons.

Questions
- Upper part of the body
  Does the person dress the upper part of the body?
  - Does the person dress the upper part of the body safely?
  - Is the right sequence used in dressing the upper part of the body?
  - How long does the person take to dress the upper part of the body?
  - What is the result of dressing the upper part of the body?
- Lower part of the body
  Does the person dress the lower part of the body?
  - Does the person dress the lower part of the body safely?
  - Is the right sequence used in dressing the lower part of the body?
  - How long does the person take to dress the lower part of the body?
  - What is the result of dressing the lower part of the body?
- Fastenings
  Does the person close fastenings?
  - Does the person close fastenings safely?
  - How long does the person take to close the fastenings?
  - Are the fastenings closed completely and in the right manner?
- Body-worn aids
  Does the person apply body-worn aids?
  - Does the person apply body-worn aids safely?
  - Does the person apply the aids in a right sequence?
  - How long does the person take to apply the aids?
  - Are the aids correctly applied?
- Ornaments/adornments
  Does the person put on ornaments or adornments?
  - Does the person put on ornaments or adornments safely?
  - Does the person put ornaments or adornments on in the right sequence?
  - How long does the person take to put on ornaments/adornments?
  - What is the result of putting ornaments/adornments on?

Undressing

Item description
'*Undressing*' comprises the actual undressing and the putting aside of the clothes (for instance in a wardrobe or on a chair). Also the removal of body-worn aids and ornaments/adornments are assessed under this item.

Sub-item description
- Upper part of the body
  Assessment is made of undressing and putting aside of the clothes of the upper part of the body. This concerns the head, the upper extremities and the upper part of the trunk. This sub-item assesses the taking off of a blouse or a sweater, gloves, a hat and so on. The kind of clothes may influence the score. For instance, the person takes off summer-wear quite easily but needs help with a heavy winter-overcoat. *Excluding*: the opening of fastenings. This is assessed under the sub-item '*fastenings*'.
- Lower part of the body
  Assessment is made of the undressing and putting aside of the clothes of the lower part of the body. This concerns the lower part of the trunk and the lower extremities. This sub-item assesses the taking off of pants, panty-hoses, shoes and so on. The kind of clothes may influence the score. For instance, the person takes off pants quite easily but needs help with a panty-hose. *Excluding*: the opening of fastenings. This is assessed under the sub-item '*fastenings*'.
- Fastenings
  Assessment is made of the opening of fastenings. This sub-item assesses zip-fasteners, bra-fastenings, boot-laces, buttons and suspenders.
- Body-worn aids
  Assessment is made of the taking off and putting aside of body-worn aids like splints, orthoses and protheses. Also the handling of glasses, contact lenses and, dentures are assessed under this sub-item.
- Ornaments/adornments
  Assessment is made of the taking off and putting aside of ornaments or adornments like rings, chains and watches.

Criteria for judgement
- Safety during undressing.
- The sequence of actions during undressing.
- The speed of undressing.
- The result of undressing.

Questions
- Upper part of the body

  Does the person undress the upper part of the body?
  - Does the person undress the upper part of the body safely?
  - Is the right sequence used in undressing the upper part of the body?
  - How long does the person take to undress the upper part of the body?
  - What is the result of undressing the upper part of the body?
- Lower part of the body

  Does the person undress the lower part of the body?
  - Does the person undress the lower part of the body safely?
  - Is the right sequence used in undressing the lower part of the body?
  - How long does the person take to undress the lower part of the body?
  - What is the result of undressing the lower part of the body?
- Fastenings

  Does the person open fastenings?
  - Does the person open fastenings safely?
  - How long does the person take to open the fastenings?
  - Are the fastenings opened completely and in the right manner?
- Body-worn aids

  Does the person remove body-worn aids?
  - Does the person remove body-worn aids safely?
  - Does the person take off the aids in a right sequence?
  - How long does the person take to remove the aids?
  - Are the aids correctly removed?
- Ornaments/adornment

  Does the person remove ornaments or adornments?
  - Does the person remove ornaments or adornments safely?
  - Does the person remove ornaments or adornments in the right sequence?
  - How long does the person take to remove ornaments/adornments?
  - What is the result of removing ornaments/adornments?

Maintaining continence

Item description
Maintaining continence comprises all actions connected with the maintenance of continence. This concerns the timely reaching of the lavatory or continence materials, undressing and dressing, being seated on the lavatory or the placing of continence materials, hygiene and removal or flushing.

Sub-item description
- Reaching in time
Assessment is made of the timely reaching of the lavatory or the incontinence materials.
- (Un)dressing
Assessment is made of the undressing and dressing of body parts which are relevant for the maintenance of continence.
- Being seated/placing
Assessment is made of the actions of sitting on and rising from the lavatory or the handling of the bedpan, the urinal, the insertion of a catheter, uritip or a stoma bag. Also the transfer from wheelchair to lavatory and vice versa is assessed under this sub-item.
- Hygiene
Assessment is made of the maintenance of hygiene during and after the defecation and urinating (for instance, handling toilet paper). Also the handling of continence materials is assessed.
- Removing/flushing
Assessment is made of the flushing of the defecation and urine or the emptying and washing of the urinal or bedpan, the removal and throwing away of a catheter or stoma bag.

Criteria for judgement
- Safety during maintenance of continence.
- The sequence of the actions during maintenance of continence.
- The speed of maintaining continence.
- The result of maintaining continence.

Questions

- Reaching in time
  Does the person reach the lavatory or the incontinence materials in time?
  - Does the person reach the lavatory or the incontinence materials safely?
- (Un)dressing
  Does the person undress and dress?
  - Does the person undress and dress safely?
  - Does the person act in the right sequences during undressing and dressing?
  - How long does undressing and dressing take?
  - What is the result of undressing and dressing (for instance: are clothes sufficiently removed)?
- Being seated/placing
  Does the person sit down and rise from the toilet?
  Does the person place the continence materials?
  - Does the person sit down and rise from the toilet or place the continence materials safely?
  - Does the person act in the right sequence?
  - How long does the person take to sit down or place the continence materials?
  - What is the result of being seated or placing (for instance: the person places the continence material wrongly)?
- Hygiene
  Does the person maintain the hygiene?
  - Does the person maintain the hygiene safely?
  - Does the person act in the right sequence?
  - How long does the person take to maintain the hygiene?
  - What is the result of maintaining the hygiene?
- Removing/flushing
  Does the person remove/flush the excretion products?
  - Does the person remove/flush the excretion products safely?
  - Does the person act in the right sequence?
  - How long does the person take to remove/flush the products?
  - What is the result of removal/flushing (for instance: are the resources (e.g. the toilet) clean)?

Providing for meals

Item description
'Providing for meals' comprises shopping, handling of food and drinks (for instance cutting up, peeling and handling packaging and kitchen utensils), cooking (for instance baking, frying and handling requisite kitchen utensils), serving and clearing of the table and hygiene (for instance washing up and cleaning the kitchen utensils). *Excluding*: the preparing of food and drinks just before eating and the actual eating and drinking. This is assessed in the domain *'personal care'* under the item *'eating and drinking'*.

Sub-item description
- Shopping
  Assessment is made of shopping and the transport of the purchases to home. Shopping includes the drawing up of a shopping list, handling of the shopping trolley, dealing with money and so on.
- Handling food
  Assessment is made of the handling of food and drinks. This concerns handling packaging and kitchen utensils but also the weighing, mixing, washing, cutting up, peeling, greasing and so on. Making coffee or tea is also assessed under this sub-item.
- Cooking food
  Assessment is made of cooking, baking, frying, grilling and handling the requisite kitchen utensils (for instance: a frying-pan, heat-resistant dish or (microwave oven).
- Serving food
  Assessment is made of the serving of food and drinks. This concerns activities like setting the table, carrying the dishes and serving tray, serving and pouring out food and so on. Clearing the table is also assessed under this sub-item.
- Hygiene
  Assessment is made of the cleaning of machines and kitchen utensils used for preparing, handling food and the actual eating and drinking. This concerns activities like washing up, drying off, putting away of kitchen-utensils, throwing away left-overs and so on.

Criteria for judgement
- Safety during providing for meals.
- The sequence of actions during providing for meals.
- The result of providing for meals.
- How long does it take to provide for meals?
- The frequency of providing for meals.

Questions
- Shopping
  Does the person do the shopping?
  - Does the person do the shopping safely?
  - Is the sequence in shopping adequate?
  - What is the result of shopping?
  - How long does person take to do the shopping?
- Handling food
  Does the person handle food and drinks?
  - Does the person handle food and drinks safely?
  - Is the sequence in handling adequate (for instance, first weighing and then mixing the ingredients)?
  - What is the result of handling food and drinks? (for instance are the packages opened sufficiently, are the vegetables well rinsed and peeled)?
  - How long does person take to handle food and drinks?
- Cooking food
  Does the person cook?
  - Does the person cook safely?
  - Is the sequence in cooking adequate (for instance, concerning handling kitchen utensils)?
  - What is the result of cooking?
  - How long does person take to cook?
- Serving food
  Does the person serve and clean up after eating and drinking?
  - Does the person serve and clean up after eating and drinking safely (for instance, not too heavy serving trays)?
  - Is the sequence in serving food adequate?
  - What is the result of serving food?
  - How long does person take to serve food?
- Hygiene
  Does the person take care of hygiene after the eating and drinking?
  - Does the person take care of hygiene after the eating and drinking safely?
  - Is the sequence in the maintenance of hygiene adequate?
  - What is the result of the maintenance of hygiene?
  - How long does person take to maintain hygiene?

Household activities

Item description
'*Household activities*' comprises the looking after and maintenance of the interior of the house. This concerns making the bed, cleaning the house (by hand or machine) and doing the laundry.

Sub-item description
- Making the bed
  Assessment is made of making the bed.
- Cleaning
  Assessment is made of the cleaning of the house. This concerns activities done by hand as well as those by machine. This concerns, for instance, dusting, sweeping the floor, washing the floor, cleaning the windows, vacuum cleaning, polishing and scrubbing.
- Doing the laundry
  Assessment is made of doing the washing and making use of the requisite apparatus. This concerns, for instance, doing small washes (hand washes), the main wash, hanging out the wash, drying, ironing, folding up and putting away. Requisite apparatus are, for instance, a washing-machine, spin-drier and an iron.

Criteria for judgement
- Safety.
- The sequence of the actions in household activities.
- The result of the household activities.
- The time span of the household activities.

Questions
- Making the bed
Does the person make the bed?
    - Does the person make the bed safely (for instance: airing the blankets/quilt)?
    - What is the sequence in making the bed like?
    - How long does it take to make the bed?
    - What is the result of making the bed?
- Cleaning
Does the person clean the house?
    - Does the person clean the house safely (for instance: while using machines)?
    - What is the sequence in cleaning like?
    - How long does the cleaning take?
    - What is the result of cleaning?
- Doing the laundry
Does the person do the laundry?
    - Does the person do the laundry safely (for instance: while using a washing-machine)?
    - What is the sequence in doing the laundry like?
    - How long does it take to do the laundry?
    - What is the result of doing the laundry?

Professional activities

Item description
'Professional activities' comprises education, daily routine, the work performance and the relation with colleagues during the practise of a profession. Participation in household activities are also assessed under this item.

Sub-item description
- Education
  Assessment is made of attendance in any form of course. This also includes education to enable the person to practise a profession (again): retraining.
- Daily routine
  Assessment is made of the adaptation of the person to the rules and standard procedures applicable to certain situations, for instance rules concerning being on time, keeping agreements and so on.
- Work performance
  Assessment is made of the person's performance. Both qualitative (adequacy, efficiency, effectiveness) and quantitative (quantity and frequency of the work results) aspects are taken into account.
- Contact with colleagues
  Assessment is made of the contact the person has with other people in the scope of work.

Criteria for judgement
- Education
  - Organizing education.
  - The required routine.
  - The result of the education.
- Daily routine
  - Presence at work.
  - Being on time at work.
  - Dealing with the rules at work.
  - Organizing the work.
  - The regularity of the work.
- Work performance
  - Getting the work done in time.
  - The result of the work.
- Contact with colleagues
  - The relationship with colleagues at work.
  - Discord at work.
  - The settling of discord at work.

Questions

- Education
  Does the person attend any form of education?
  - Has the person recently attended the courses regularly?
  - Are the results sufficient?
- Daily routine
  Does the person have difficulty with the daily routine at work?
  - Does the person get to work on time?
  - How does the person deal with rules at work?
  - Does the person succeed in organizing his or her work adequately?
  - Does the person have difficulties with the required regularity?
- Work performance
  What is the person's work performance like?
  - Is the work delivered on time?
  - Has the work recently been too much for the person?
  - What are the results of the work like?
  - Has there recently been any criticism from others concerning the person's work performance?
- Contact with colleagues
  What are the contacts with colleagues like?
  - How frequent are these contacts?
  - Are there often disagreements or discord?
  - Has discord at work been settled?

Leisure activities

Item description
'Leisure activities' comprises pastimes/hobbies and sport.

Sub-item description
- Pastimes/hobbies
  Assessment is made of the presence of pastimes/hobbies like painting, computer hobbies, watching tv, doing needlework, knitting, playing music, puzzling, keeping animals, gardening and so on, as well as attending recreational courses.
- Sport
  Assessment is made of the participation in some kind of sport. It is of no concern whether the sport is practised recreationally, professionally, individually or as a team.

Criteria for judgement
- Safety during the leisure activities.
- The sequence of actions during the leisure activities.
- The pace of the leisure activities.
- Dealing with the rules during leisure activities.

Questions
- Pastimes/hobbies
Does the person have any pastimes/hobbies?
  - Are the pastimes/hobbies practised in a safe way?
  - What is the sequence of actions like during the pastimes/hobbies?
  - What is the pace like during the pastimes/hobbies?
- Sport
Does the person practise any kind of sport?
  - Does the person practise any kind of sport safely?
  - What is the sequence of actions like during the practise of the sport?
  - What is the pace like during the sport?
  - How does the person deal with the rules of the games?

Partner

Item description
'Partner' comprises the continuation of the relation with the partner, as existing before the disease or disorder. Relation comprises roles, emotional ties, the undertaking of activities together and the sexual relationship with the partner.

Sub-item description
- Role
  Assessment is made of the continuation of the role arrangement, just as it existed before the disease or disorder, between the person and the partner. This sub-item concerns roles such as: the role as caretaker, dependent role, role as father, and role as mother.
- Emotional ties
  Assessment is made of the continuation of the affective relationship with the partner, just as it existed before the disease or disorder. This concerns the communication between each other (talking about the disease or disorder, the children, the news and daily events) and the presence of mutual feelings of respect, trust and affection.
- Activities
  Assessment is made of the continuation of undertaking social and cultural activities together (for instance, dining together, visiting relatives, visiting the theater and such) and taking care of the partner, just as existing before the disease or disorder.
- Sexual relation
  Assessment is made of the continuation of the sexual relationship with the sexual partner (heterosexual or homosexual), just as this was before the disease or disorder. The nature of the sexual activities has no influence on the score.

Criteria for judgement
- Role
  - Decision-taking.
  - Mutual role distribution.
  - Wage-earning relationship.
  - Doing household activities.
- Emotional ties
  - Mutual intimacy.
  - Way of communicating with each other.
  - Criticizing each other.
  - The presence of disagreements.

- Activities
  - Going out.
  - Taking care of the partner.
- Sexual relation
  - Frequency of sexual relations.
  - Satisfaction concerning the sexual relationship.
  - Difficulties in the sexual relationship.

Questions

- Role
  Has the role distribution between the person and the partner been changed by the disorder?
  - Who takes the important decisions?
  - Who has the role as caretaker?
  - Who has the role as wage-earner?
  - Who is doing the household activities?
- Emotional ties
  Has the emotional tie with the partner been changed by the disorder?
  - Has the intimacy with the partner changed?
  - Does the person talk in the same way (as before the disorder) on subjects with his or her partner?
  - Does the partner criticize the person more often in the period in question?
  - Have there been more disagreements or quarrels?
- Activities
  Has the undertaking of social and cultural activities been changed by the disorder?
  - Has the pattern of going out changed?
  - Has anything changed in the care for the partner?
- Sexual relation
  Has the sexual relationship with the partner been changed by the disorder?
  - Has anything changed in the frequency or satisfaction?
  - Have there been problems in the sexual relationship in the period in question?
  - Are these caused by the disorder?

Child(ren)

Item description
'Child(ren)' comprises the continuation of the relationship with the person's own children, just as existed before the disease or disorder. This concerns the role distribution, the emotional ties and the activities concerned with upbringing, taking care and doing other activities together. The item concerns children living at home as well as those living elsewhere.

Sub-item description
- Role
  Assessment is made of the continuation of the role distribution, just as this was before the disorder between the person and child(ren). Role covers: the role as caretaker, as father or mother and suchlike.
- Emotional ties
  Assessment is made of the continuation of the affective relationship with the children as expressed by mutual feelings of respect, trust and affection.
- Activities
  Assessment is made of the continuation of the contribution of the person in the upbringing and caring (for instance, feeding, putting to bed, bringing to school) of the children and/or the undertaking of activities together (for instance, playing games, reading stories, watching TV, outings).

Criteria for judgement
- Role
  - Decision-taking.
  - Mutual role distribution.
- Emotional ties
  - The presence of respect.
  - Way of communicating.
  - Criticizing each other.
  - The presence of disagreements.
- Activities
  - Contribution to the upbringing.
  - Undertaking outings.

Questions

- Role

  Has the role distribution between the person and his or her child(ren) been changed by the disorder?
  - Who takes the important decisions?
  - Who has the caring role?

- Emotional ties

  Have the emotional ties with the children been changed by the disorder?
  - Do the children still respect the person?
  - Does the person talk on the same subjects openly with his or her children?
  - Do the children criticize the person more in the period in question than before the disorder?
  - Have disagreements or quarrels become more frequent? Have these been settled?

- Activities

  Has the undertaking of activities together with the children been changed by the disorder?
  - Does the person in the same way contribute to bringing up the children?
  - Does the person go on outings with the children?

Friends/acquaintances

Item description
'Friends/acquaintances' comprises the continuation of the relationship with friends and acquaintances, just as this was before the disorder. This covers the emotional ties, the activities together and, if applicable, the continuation of participation in social groups, organizations or unions.

Sub-item description
- Emotional ties
  Assessment is made of the continuation of the affective relationship with friends or acquaintances, as expressed in mutual trust and emotional support. This sub-item comprises also the contacts the person has through participation in social groups, organizations or unions.
- Activities
  Assessment is made of the continuation of the activities with friends or acquaintances, just like those that took place before the disorder.

Criteria for judgement
- Emotional ties
  - Frequency of visits.
  - Way of communicating.
  - Criticizing each other.
  - The presence of disagreements.
- Activities
  - Participating in activities.

Questions
- Emotional ties

  Has the relationship of the person with friends or acquaintances changed?
  - Has the frequency of the visits changed?
  - Do the friends/acquaintances visit the person of their own accord?
  - Does the person talk in the same way on subjects with his or her friends?
  - Do friends (or one of them) criticize the person more in the period in question?
  - Have disagreements or quarrels become more frequent?
- Activities

  Has there been a change in the undertaking of activities with friends or acquaintances as a result of the disorder?
  - Does the person participate in the activities in the same way as before the disorder?

Score forms

The items and sub-items are included on score forms. There is one score form for the items. The five score forms for the sub-items are organized per domain. At the top of each form personal data can be noted down. Besides assigning scores for disability or handicap and the perceived problem, an additional remark on each score can be written down on the empty line behind the scores. At the bottom of each form the severity gradings and their description are mentioned.

Rehabilitation Activities Profile

Items of all domains

Name : ....

Address : ....

Post-code/zip code : ....

City : ....

Date of birth : .... Gender : m/f

Diagnosis : ....

Date : ....

Communication : .... | Disability | Problem

- Expressing : □ □ | □ □
- Comprehending : □ □ | □ □

Mobility : .... | Disability | Problem

- Maintaining posture : □ □ | □ □
- Changing posture : □ □ | □ □
- Walking : □ □ | □ □
- Using wheelchair : □ □ | □ □
- Climbing stairs : □ □ | □ □
- Using transport : □ □ | □ □

Personal care : .... | Disability | Problem

- Sleeping : □ □ | □ □
- Eating and drinking : □ □ | □ □
- Washing and grooming : □ □ | □ □
- Dressing : □ □ | □ □
- Undressing : □ □ | □ □
- Maintaining continence : □ □ | □ □

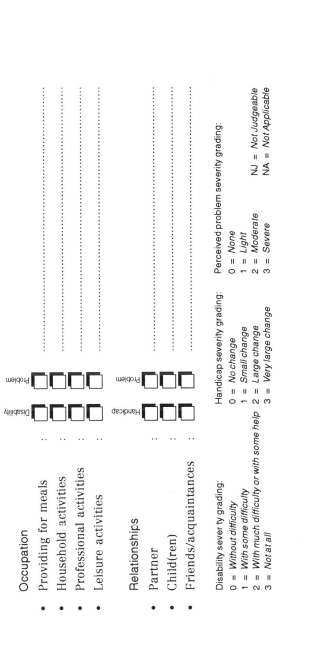

Occupation

- Providing for meals :
- Household activities :
- Professional activities :
- Leisure activities :

(Disability / Problem)

Relationships

- Partner :
- Child(ren) :
- Friends/acquaintances :

(Handicap / Problem)

Disability severity grading:
0 = *Without difficulty*
1 = *With some difficulty*
2 = *With much difficulty or with some help*
3 = *Not at all*

Handicap severity grading:
0 = *No change*
1 = *Small change*
2 = *Large change*
3 = *Very large change*

Perceived problem severity grading:
0 = *None*
1 = *Light*
2 = *Moderate*
3 = *Severe*

NJ = *Not Judgeable*
NA = *Not Applicable*

Rehabilitation Activities Profile

Sub-items of domain communication

Name : .... Date of birth : .... Gender : m/f

Address : .... Diagnosis : ....

Post-code/zip code : ....

City : .... Date : ....

	Disability	Problem
Expressing	:	....
• Nonverbal	: ☐ ☐	....
• Talking	: ☐ ☐	....
• Writing	: ☐ ☐	....
Comprehending	:	....
• Images	: ☐ ☐	....
• Sounds	: ☐ ☐	....
• Nonverbal	: ☐ ☐	....
• Spoken language	: ☐ ☐	....
• Written language	: ☐ ☐	....

Disability severity grading:

0 = *Without difficulty*
1 = *With some difficulty*
2 = *With much difficulty or with some help*
3 = *Not at all*

Perceived problem severity grading:

0 = *None*
1 = *Light*
2 = *Moderate*
3 = *Severe*

NJ = *Not Judgeable*
NA = *Not Applicable*

Rehabilitation Activities Profile

Sub-items of domain mobility

Name : .... Date of birth : .... Gender : m/f

Address : .... Diagnosis : ....

Post-code/zip code : ....

City : .... Date : ....

		Disability	Problem
Maintaining posture			
• Lying	:	▢▢▢	▢▢▢
• Sitting	:		
• Standing	:		
Changing posture			
• Lie/lie (turn around)	:	▢▢▢▢	▢▢▢▢
• Lie/sit	:		
• Sit/stand	:		
• Sit/sit-transfers	:		
Walking			
• Indoors	:	▢▢	▢▢
• Outdoors	:		
Using wheelchair			
• Indoors	:	▢▢	▢▢
• Outdoors			

Climbing stairs

- Indoors   :   □ Disability □ Problem ....
- Outdoors   :   □ Disability □ Problem ....

Using transport

- Bicycle/moped   :   □ Disability □ Problem ....
- Car   :   □ Disability □ Problem ....
- Public transport   :   □ Disability □ Problem ....
- Alternative transport   :   □ Disability □ Problem ....

Disability severity grading:

0 = Without difficulty
1 = With some difficulty
2 = With much difficulty or with some help
3 = Not at all

Perceived problem severity grading:

0 = None
1 = Light
2 = Moderate
3 = Severe

NJ = Not Judgeable
NA = Not Applicable

Rehabilitation Activities Profile

Sub-items of domain personal care

Name : ....
Address : ....
Post-code/zip code : ....
City : ....

Date of birth : ....   Gender : m/f
Diagnosis : ....

Date : ....

Sleeping   Disability | Problem
- Falling asleep : ....   ☐ ☐ | ☐ ☐
- Sleeping on : ....

Eating and drinking   Disability | Problem
- Preparing food : ....   ☐ ☐ ☐ | ☐ ☐ ☐
- Conveying food to mouth : ....
- Chewing/swallowing : ....

Washing and grooming   Disability | Problem
- Face and hair : ....   ☐ ☐ ☐ | ☐ ☐ ☐
- Upper part of the body : ....
- Lower part of the body : ....

Dressing   Disability | Problem
- Upper part of the body : ....   ☐ ☐ ☐ ☐ ☐ | ☐ ☐ ☐ ☐ ☐
- Lower part of the body : ....
- Fastenings : ....
- Body-worn aids : ....
- Ornaments/adornments :

Undressing

	Disability	Problem	
• Upper part of the body	:	☐ ☐	....
• Lower part of the body	:	☐ ☐	....
• Fastenings	:	☐ ☐	....
• Body-worn aids	:	☐ ☐	....
• Ornaments/adornments	:	☐ ☐	....

Maintaining continence

	Disability	Problem	
• Reaching in time	:	☐ ☐	....
• (Un)dressing	:	☐ ☐	....
• Being seated/placing	:	☐ ☐	....
• Hygiene	:	☐ ☐	....
• Removing/flushing	:	☐ ☐	....

Disability severity grading:

0 = *Without difficulty*
1 = *With some difficulty*
2 = *With much difficulty or with some help*
3 = *Not at all*

Perceived problem severity grading:

0 = *None*
1 = *Light*
2 = *Moderate*
3 = *Severe*

NJ = *Not Judgeable*
NA = *Not Applicable*

Rehabilitation Activities Profile

Sub-items of domain occupation

Name : ....

Address : ....

Post-code/zip code : ....

City : ....

Date of birth : .... Gender : m/f

Diagnosis : ....

Date : ....

Providing for meals   Disability   Problem

- Shopping : ☐☐☐☐☐   ☐☐☐☐☐
- Handling food :
- Cooking food :
- Serving food :
- Hygiene :

....

....

....

....

....

Household activities   Disability   Problem

- Making the bed : ☐☐☐   ☐☐☐
- Cleaning :
- Doing the laundry :

....

....

....

Professional activities   Disability   Problem

- Education : ☐☐☐☐   ☐☐☐☐
- Daily routine :
- Work performance :
- Contact with colleagues :

....

....

....

....

Leisure activities

- Pastimes/hobbies   :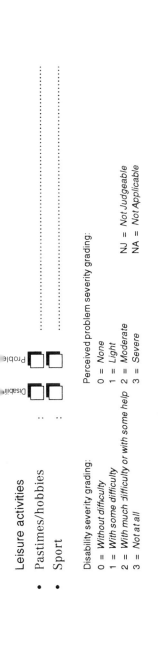
- Sport   :

Disability severity grading:

0 = *Without difficulty*
1 = *With some difficulty*
2 = *With much difficulty or with some help*
3 = *Not at all*

Perceived problem severity grading:

0 = *None*
1 = *Light*
2 = *Moderate*
3 = *Severe*

NJ = *Not Judgeable*
NA = *Not Applicable*

Rehabilitation Activities Profile

Sub-items of domain relationships

Name : .... Date of birth : .... Gender : m/f

Address : .... Diagnosis : ....

Post-code/zip code : ....

City : .... Date : ....

	Handicap	Problem	
Partner			
• Role	:	☐☐☐☐ / ☐☐☐☐	....
• Emotional ties	:		....
• Activities	:		....
• Sexual relation	:		....
Child(ren)			
• Role	:	☐☐☐ / ☐☐☐	....
• Emotional ties	:		....
• Activities	:		....
Friends/acquaintances			
• Emotional ties	:	☐☐ / ☐☐	....
• Activities	:		....

Handicap severity grading:

0 = No change
1 = Small change
2 = Large change
3 = Very large change

Perceived problem severity grading:

0 = None
1 = Light
2 = Moderate
3 = Severe

NJ = Not Judgeable
NA = Not Applicable